MY ESSENTIAL OIL RECIPES

THIS BOOK BELONGS TO

_____

_____

_____

CONTACT DETAILS

_____

_____

_____

_____

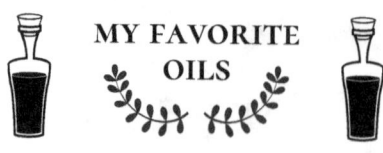

MY FAVORITE OILS

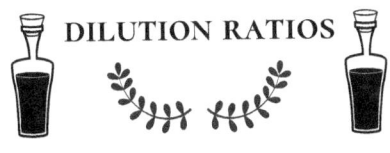

DILUTION RATIOS

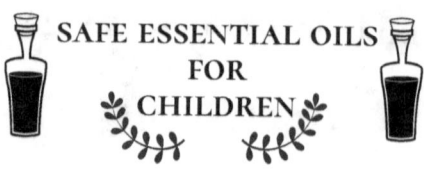

SAFE ESSENTIAL OILS
FOR
CHILDREN

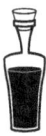 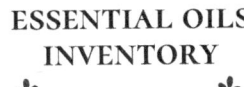 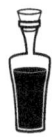

ESSENTIAL OILS INVENTORY

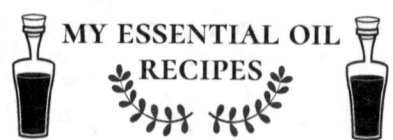

MY ESSENTIAL OIL RECIPES

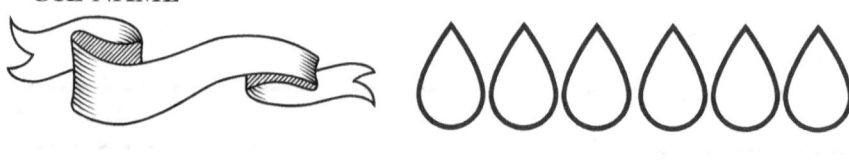

OIL NAME

BENEFITS

_____

_____

_____

_____

NOTES

_____

_____

_____

_____

OIL NAME

BENEFITS

_____

_____

_____

_____

NOTES

_____

_____

_____

_____

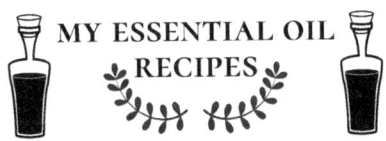

MY ESSENTIAL OIL RECIPES

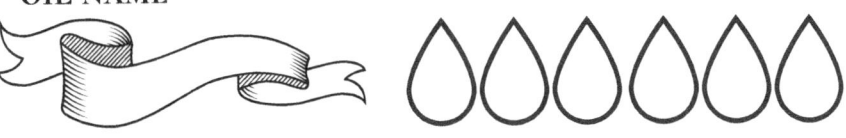

OIL NAME

BENEFITS

_____

_____

_____

_____

NOTES

_____

_____

_____

_____

OIL NAME

BENEFITS

_____

_____

_____

_____

NOTES

_____

_____

_____

_____

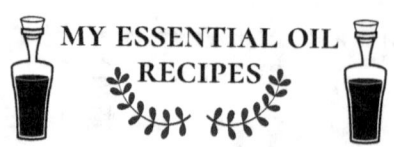

MY ESSENTIAL OIL RECIPES

OIL NAME

BENEFITS

_____

_____

_____

_____

NOTES

_____

_____

_____

_____

OIL NAME

BENEFITS

_____

_____

_____

_____

NOTES

_____

_____

_____

_____

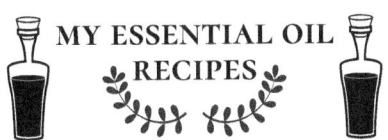

MY ESSENTIAL OIL RECIPES

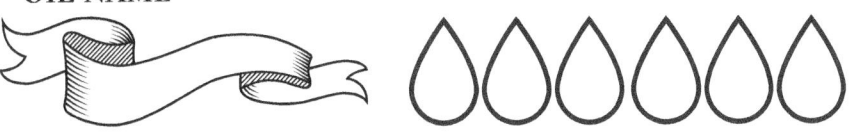

OIL NAME

BENEFITS

_____

_____

_____

_____

NOTES

_____

_____

_____

_____

OIL NAME

BENEFITS

_____

_____

_____

_____

NOTES

_____

_____

_____

_____

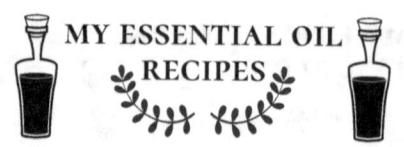

MY ESSENTIAL OIL RECIPES

OIL NAME

BENEFITS

_____
_____
_____
_____

NOTES

_____
_____
_____
_____

OIL NAME

BENEFITS

_____
_____
_____
_____

NOTES

_____
_____
_____
_____

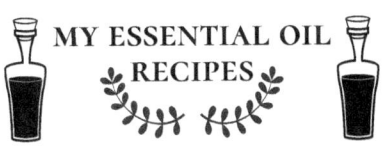

MY ESSENTIAL OIL RECIPES

OIL NAME

BENEFITS

_____

_____

_____

NOTES

_____

_____

_____

OIL NAME

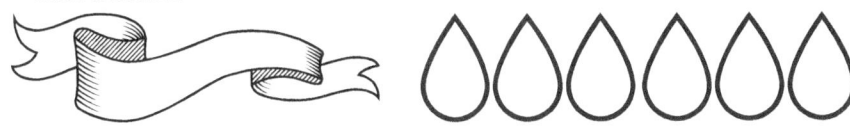

BENEFITS

_____

_____

_____

NOTES

_____

_____

_____

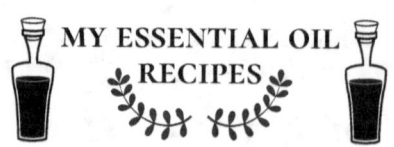

MY ESSENTIAL OIL RECIPES

OIL NAME

BENEFITS

NOTES

OIL NAME

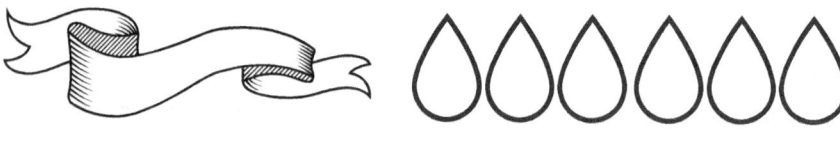

BENEFITS

NOTES

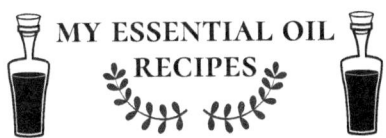

MY ESSENTIAL OIL RECIPES

OIL NAME

BENEFITS

_____

_____

_____

NOTES

_____

_____

_____

OIL NAME

BENEFITS

_____

_____

_____

NOTES

_____

_____

_____

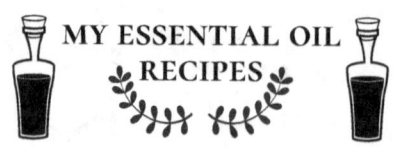

MY ESSENTIAL OIL RECIPES

OIL NAME

BENEFITS

_____

_____

_____

_____

NOTES

_____

_____

_____

_____

OIL NAME

BENEFITS

_____

_____

_____

_____

NOTES

_____

_____

_____

_____

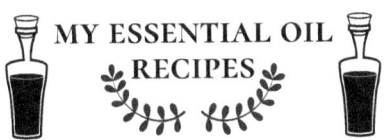

MY ESSENTIAL OIL RECIPES

OIL NAME

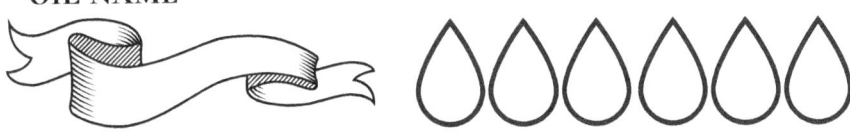

BENEFITS

_____

_____

_____

_____

NOTES

_____

_____

_____

_____

OIL NAME

BENEFITS

_____

_____

_____

_____

NOTES

_____

_____

_____

_____

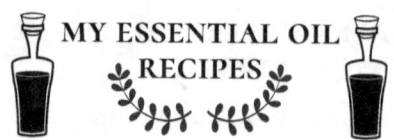

MY ESSENTIAL OIL RECIPES

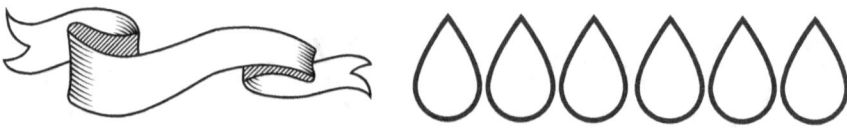

OIL NAME

BENEFITS

_____

_____

_____

_____

NOTES

_____

_____

_____

_____

OIL NAME

BENEFITS

_____

_____

_____

_____

NOTES

_____

_____

_____

_____

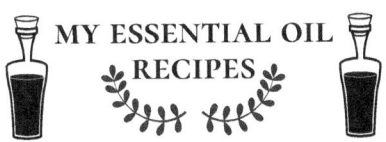

MY ESSENTIAL OIL RECIPES

OIL NAME

BENEFITS

_____

_____

_____

NOTES

_____

_____

_____

_____

OIL NAME

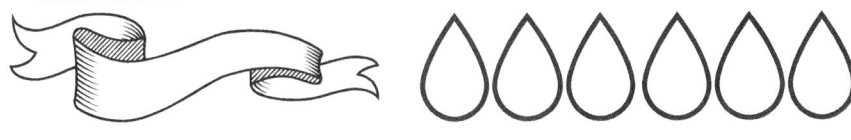

BENEFITS

_____

_____

_____

NOTES

_____

_____

_____

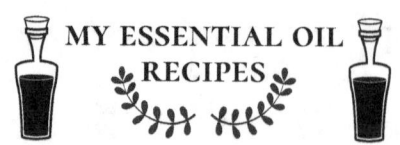

MY ESSENTIAL OIL RECIPES

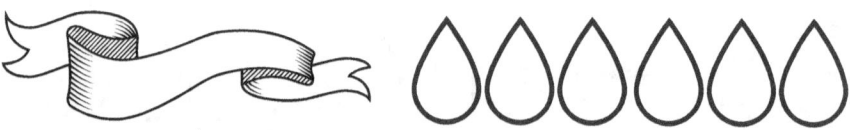

OIL NAME

BENEFITS

NOTES

OIL NAME

BENEFITS

NOTES

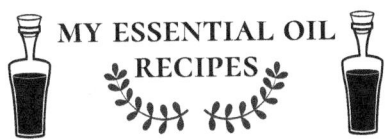

MY ESSENTIAL OIL RECIPES

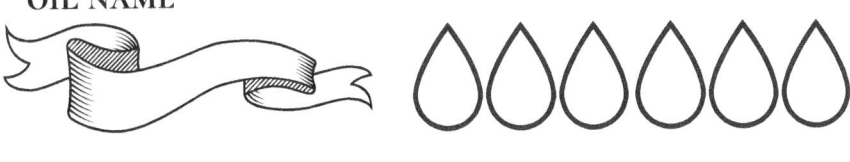

OIL NAME

BENEFITS

_____

_____

_____

_____

NOTES

_____

_____

_____

_____

OIL NAME

BENEFITS

_____

_____

_____

_____

NOTES

_____

_____

_____

_____

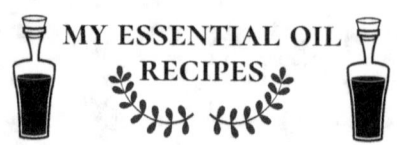

MY ESSENTIAL OIL RECIPES

OIL NAME

BENEFITS

_____

_____

_____

_____

NOTES

_____

_____

_____

_____

OIL NAME

BENEFITS

_____

_____

_____

_____

NOTES

_____

_____

_____

_____

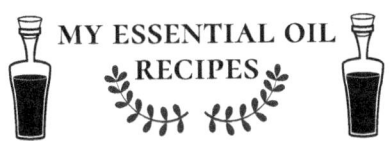

MY ESSENTIAL OIL RECIPES

OIL NAME

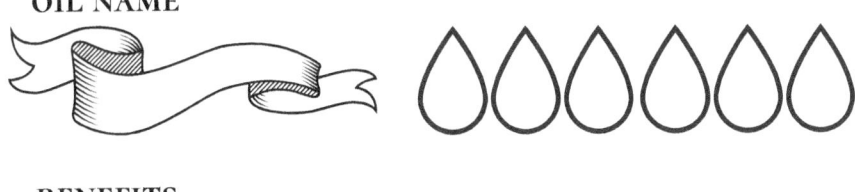

BENEFITS

_____

_____

_____

NOTES

_____

_____

_____

OIL NAME

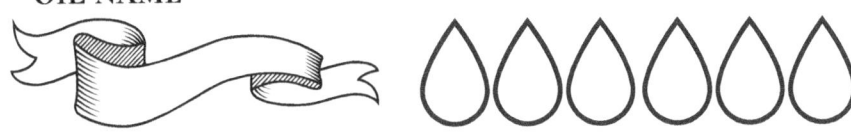

BENEFITS

_____

_____

_____

NOTES

_____

_____

_____

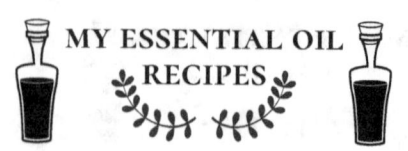

MY ESSENTIAL OIL RECIPES

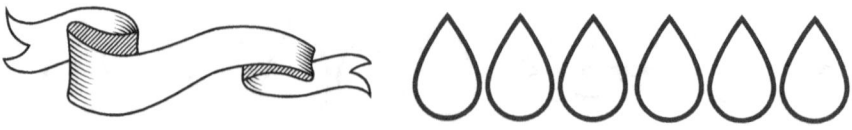

OIL NAME

BENEFITS

NOTES

OIL NAME

BENEFITS

NOTES

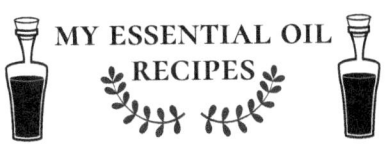

MY ESSENTIAL OIL RECIPES

OIL NAME

BENEFITS

_____

_____

_____

NOTES

_____

_____

_____

OIL NAME

BENEFITS

_____

_____

_____

NOTES

_____

_____

_____

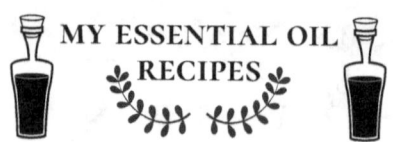

MY ESSENTIAL OIL RECIPES

OIL NAME

BENEFITS

_____

_____

_____

_____

NOTES

_____

_____

_____

OIL NAME

BENEFITS

_____

_____

_____

_____

NOTES

_____

_____

_____

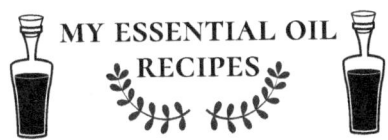

MY ESSENTIAL OIL RECIPES

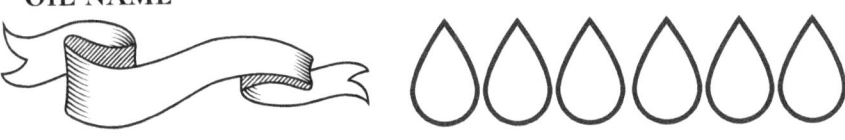

OIL NAME

BENEFITS

NOTES

OIL NAME

BENEFITS

NOTES

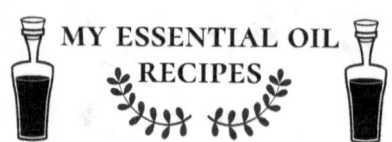

MY ESSENTIAL OIL RECIPES

OIL NAME

BENEFITS

_____

_____

_____

_____

NOTES

_____

_____

_____

_____

OIL NAME

BENEFITS

_____

_____

_____

_____

NOTES

_____

_____

_____

_____

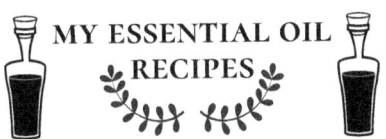

MY ESSENTIAL OIL RECIPES

OIL NAME

BENEFITS

NOTES

OIL NAME

BENEFITS

NOTES

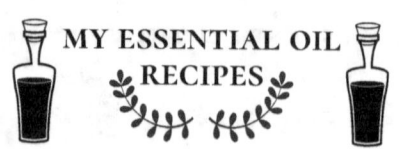

MY ESSENTIAL OIL RECIPES

OIL NAME

BENEFITS

_____

_____

_____

_____

NOTES

_____

_____

_____

_____

OIL NAME

BENEFITS

_____

_____

_____

_____

NOTES

_____

_____

_____

_____

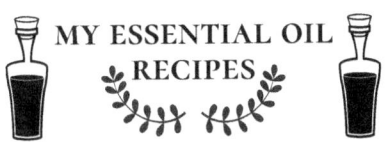

MY ESSENTIAL OIL RECIPES

OIL NAME

BENEFITS

_____

_____

_____

NOTES

_____

_____

_____

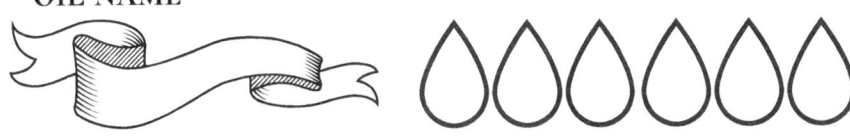

OIL NAME

BENEFITS

_____

_____

_____

NOTES

_____

_____

_____

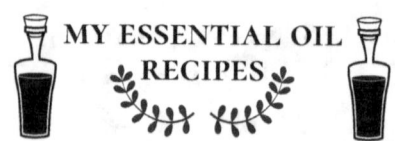

MY ESSENTIAL OIL RECIPES

OIL NAME

BENEFITS

NOTES

OIL NAME

BENEFITS

NOTES

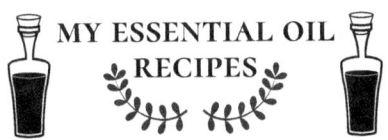

MY ESSENTIAL OIL RECIPES

OIL NAME

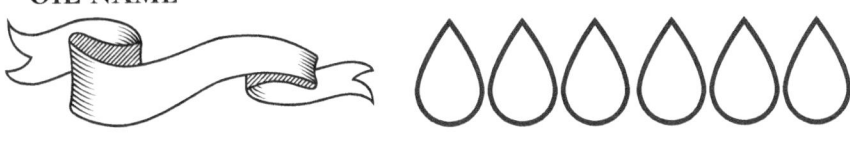

BENEFITS

_____

_____

_____

NOTES

_____

_____

_____

OIL NAME

BENEFITS

_____

_____

_____

NOTES

_____

_____

_____

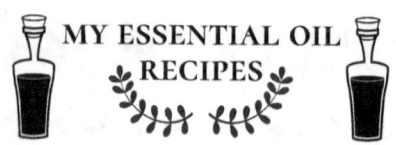

MY ESSENTIAL OIL RECIPES

OIL NAME

BENEFITS

_____

_____

_____

_____

NOTES

_____

_____

_____

_____

OIL NAME

BENEFITS

_____

_____

_____

_____

NOTES

_____

_____

_____

_____

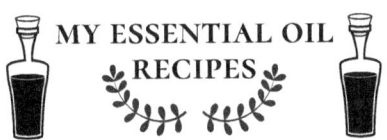

MY ESSENTIAL OIL RECIPES

OIL NAME

BENEFITS

NOTES

OIL NAME

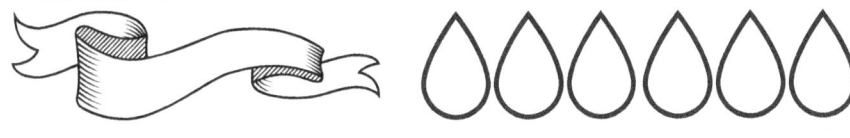

BENEFITS

NOTES

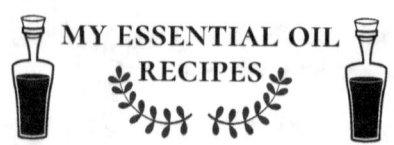

MY ESSENTIAL OIL RECIPES

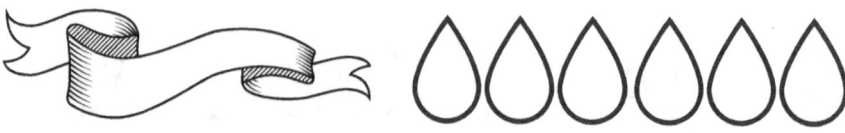

OIL NAME

BENEFITS

_____

_____

_____

_____

NOTES

_____

_____

_____

_____

OIL NAME

BENEFITS

_____

_____

_____

_____

NOTES

_____

_____

_____

_____

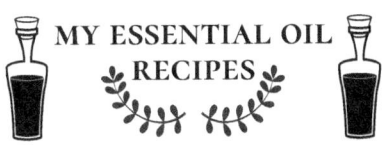

MY ESSENTIAL OIL RECIPES

OIL NAME

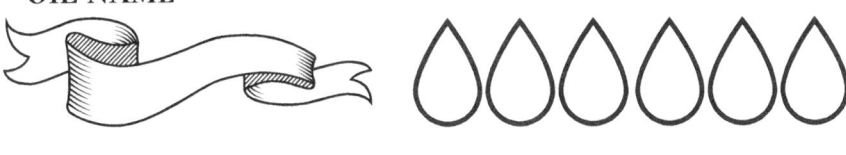

BENEFITS

_____

_____

_____

NOTES

_____

_____

_____

OIL NAME

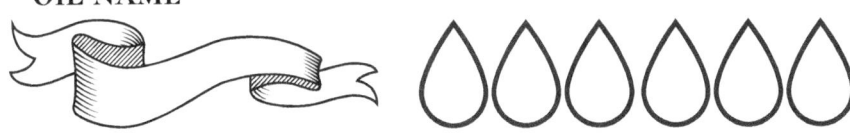

BENEFITS

_____

_____

_____

NOTES

_____

_____

_____

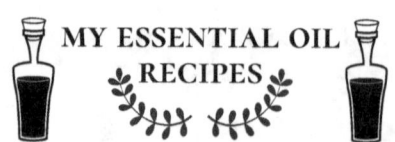

MY ESSENTIAL OIL RECIPES

OIL NAME

BENEFITS

_____
_____
_____
_____

NOTES

_____
_____
_____

OIL NAME

BENEFITS

_____
_____
_____
_____

NOTES

_____
_____
_____

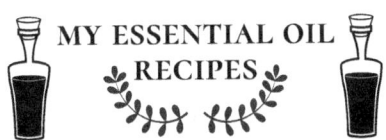

MY ESSENTIAL OIL RECIPES

OIL NAME

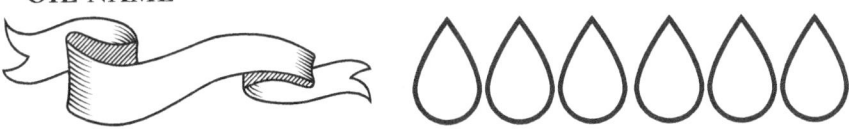

BENEFITS

_____

_____

_____

NOTES

_____

_____

_____

OIL NAME

BENEFITS

_____

_____

_____

NOTES

_____

_____

_____

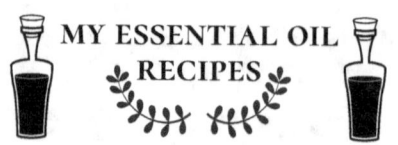

MY ESSENTIAL OIL RECIPES

OIL NAME

BENEFITS

_____
_____
_____
_____

NOTES

_____
_____
_____
_____

OIL NAME

BENEFITS

_____
_____
_____
_____

NOTES

_____
_____
_____
_____

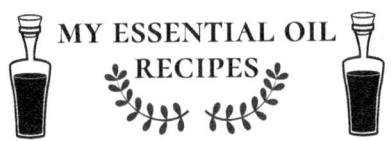

MY ESSENTIAL OIL RECIPES

OIL NAME

BENEFITS

_____

_____

_____

NOTES

_____

_____

_____

OIL NAME

BENEFITS

_____

_____

_____

NOTES

_____

_____

_____

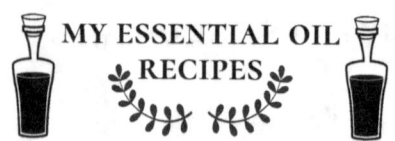

MY ESSENTIAL OIL RECIPES

OIL NAME

BENEFITS

_____

_____

_____

_____

NOTES

_____

_____

_____

_____

OIL NAME

BENEFITS

_____

_____

_____

_____

NOTES

_____

_____

_____

_____

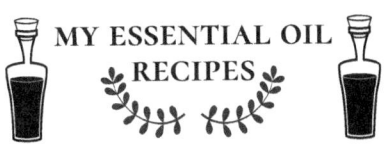

MY ESSENTIAL OIL RECIPES

OIL NAME

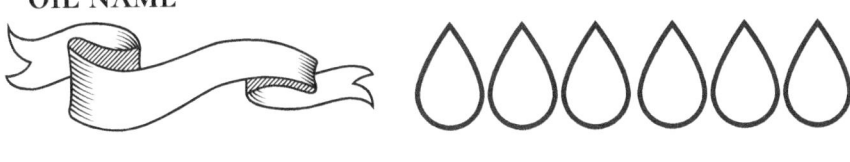

BENEFITS

_____

_____

_____

NOTES

_____

_____

_____

OIL NAME

BENEFITS

_____

_____

_____

NOTES

_____

_____

_____

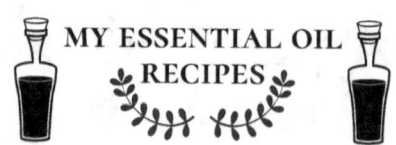

MY ESSENTIAL OIL RECIPES

OIL NAME

BENEFITS

_____
_____
_____
_____

NOTES

_____
_____
_____
_____

OIL NAME

BENEFITS

_____
_____
_____
_____

NOTES

_____
_____
_____
_____

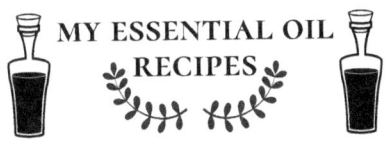

MY ESSENTIAL OIL RECIPES

OIL NAME

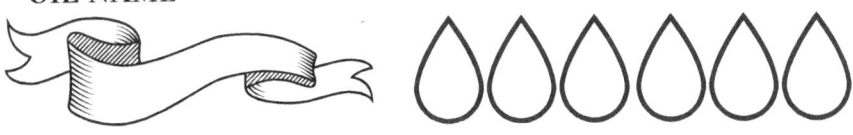

BENEFITS

_____
_____
_____
_____

NOTES

_____
_____
_____
_____

OIL NAME

BENEFITS

_____
_____
_____
_____

NOTES

_____
_____
_____
_____

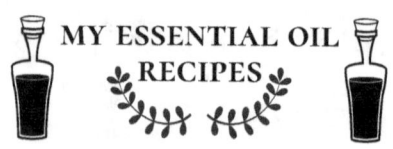

MY ESSENTIAL OIL RECIPES

OIL NAME

BENEFITS

_____

_____

_____

_____

NOTES

_____

_____

_____

_____

OIL NAME

BENEFITS

_____

_____

_____

_____

NOTES

_____

_____

_____

_____

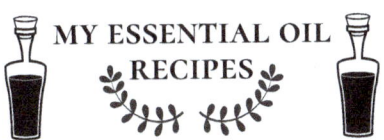

MY ESSENTIAL OIL RECIPES

OIL NAME

BENEFITS

_____
_____
_____
_____

NOTES

_____
_____
_____
_____

OIL NAME

BENEFITS

_____
_____
_____
_____

NOTES

_____
_____
_____
_____

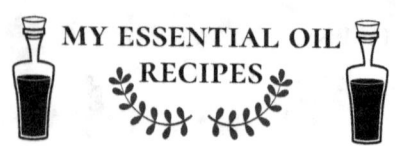

MY ESSENTIAL OIL RECIPES

OIL NAME

BENEFITS

NOTES

OIL NAME

BENEFITS

NOTES

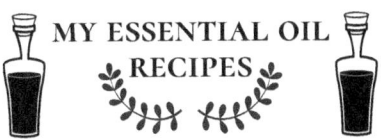

MY ESSENTIAL OIL RECIPES

OIL NAME

BENEFITS

_____

_____

_____

NOTES

_____

_____

_____

OIL NAME

BENEFITS

_____

_____

_____

NOTES

_____

_____

_____

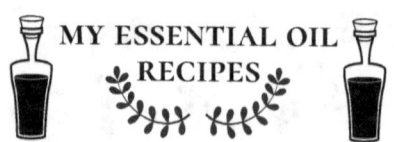

MY ESSENTIAL OIL RECIPES

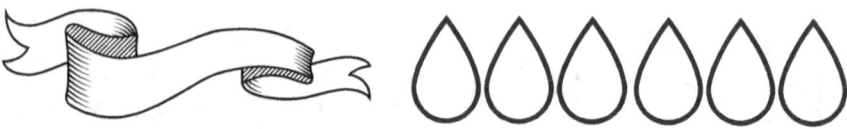

OIL NAME

BENEFITS

_____

_____

_____

_____

NOTES

_____

_____

_____

_____

OIL NAME

BENEFITS

_____

_____

_____

_____

NOTES

_____

_____

_____

_____

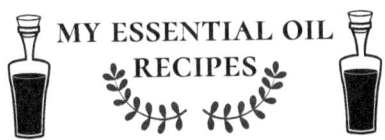

MY ESSENTIAL OIL RECIPES

OIL NAME

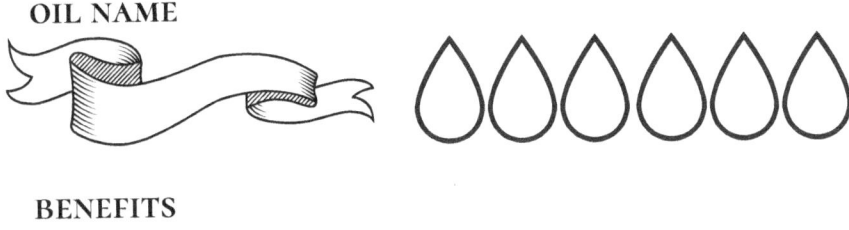

BENEFITS

_____

_____

_____

_____

NOTES

_____

_____

_____

_____

OIL NAME

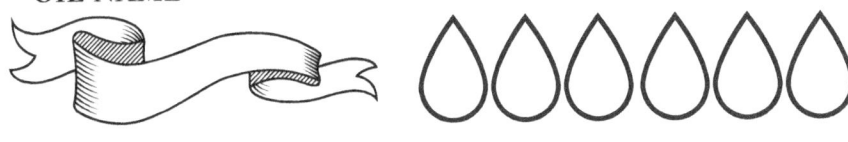

BENEFITS

_____

_____

_____

_____

NOTES

_____

_____

_____

_____

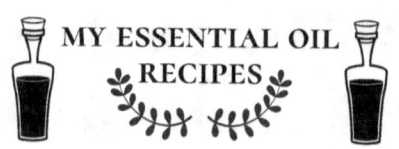

MY ESSENTIAL OIL RECIPES

OIL NAME

BENEFITS

_____

_____

_____

_____

NOTES

_____

_____

_____

_____

OIL NAME

BENEFITS

_____

_____

_____

_____

NOTES

_____

_____

_____

_____

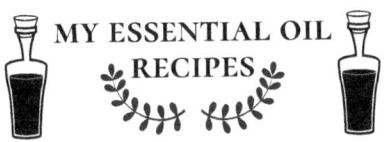

MY ESSENTIAL OIL RECIPES

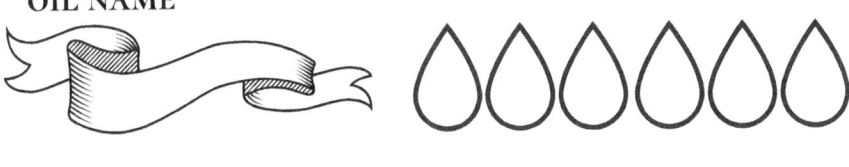

OIL NAME

BENEFITS

_____

_____

_____

_____

NOTES

_____

_____

_____

OIL NAME

BENEFITS

_____

_____

_____

_____

NOTES

_____

_____

_____

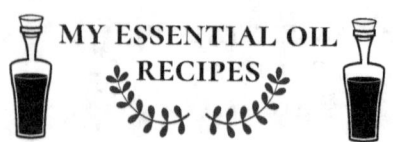

MY ESSENTIAL OIL RECIPES

OIL NAME

BENEFITS

NOTES

OIL NAME

BENEFITS

NOTES

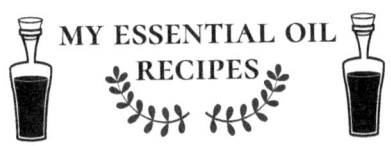

MY ESSENTIAL OIL RECIPES

OIL NAME

BENEFITS

_____

_____

_____

_____

NOTES

_____

_____

_____

_____

OIL NAME

BENEFITS

_____

_____

_____

_____

NOTES

_____

_____

_____

_____

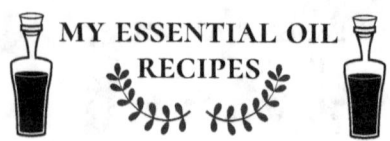

MY ESSENTIAL OIL RECIPES

OIL NAME

BENEFITS

_____

_____

_____

_____

NOTES

_____

_____

_____

_____

OIL NAME

BENEFITS

_____

_____

_____

_____

NOTES

_____

_____

_____

_____

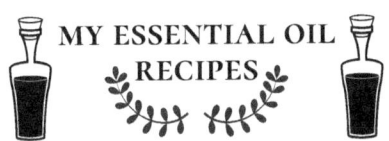

MY ESSENTIAL OIL RECIPES

OIL NAME

BENEFITS

_____

_____

_____

NOTES

_____

_____

_____

OIL NAME

BENEFITS

_____

_____

_____

NOTES

_____

_____

_____

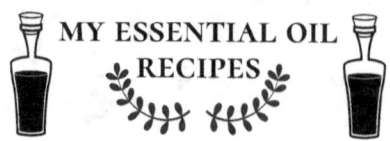

MY ESSENTIAL OIL RECIPES

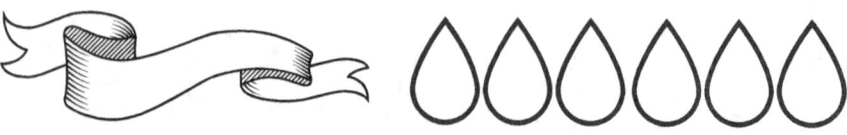

OIL NAME

BENEFITS

_____

_____

_____

_____

NOTES

_____

_____

_____

_____

OIL NAME

BENEFITS

_____

_____

_____

_____

NOTES

_____

_____

_____

_____

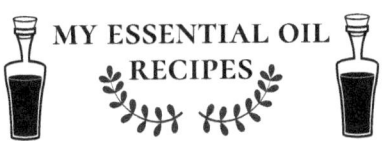
MY ESSENTIAL OIL RECIPES

OIL NAME

BENEFITS

_____
_____
_____
_____

NOTES

_____
_____
_____
_____

OIL NAME

BENEFITS

_____
_____
_____
_____

NOTES

_____
_____
_____
_____

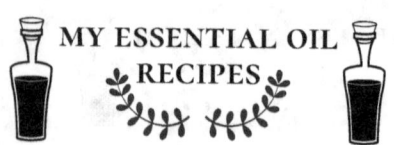

MY ESSENTIAL OIL RECIPES

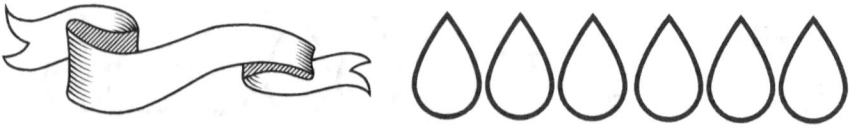

OIL NAME

BENEFITS

_____

_____

_____

_____

NOTES

_____

_____

_____

_____

OIL NAME

BENEFITS

_____

_____

_____

_____

NOTES

_____

_____

_____

_____

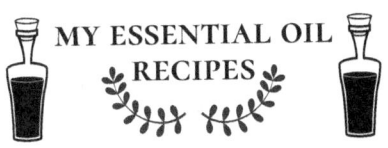

MY ESSENTIAL OIL RECIPES

OIL NAME

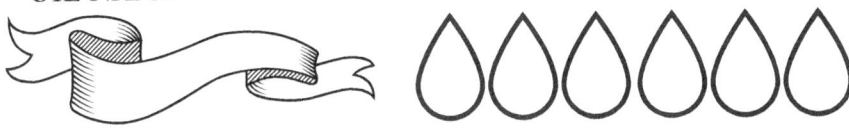

BENEFITS

_____

_____

_____

_____

NOTES

_____

_____

_____

OIL NAME

BENEFITS

_____

_____

_____

_____

NOTES

_____

_____

_____

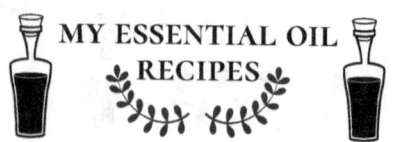

MY ESSENTIAL OIL RECIPES

OIL NAME

BENEFITS

_____

_____

_____

_____

NOTES

_____

_____

_____

_____

OIL NAME

BENEFITS

_____

_____

_____

_____

NOTES

_____

_____

_____

_____

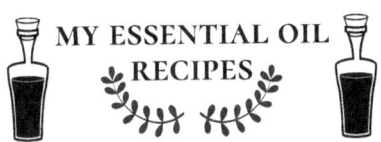

MY ESSENTIAL OIL RECIPES

OIL NAME

BENEFITS

_____

_____

_____

NOTES

_____

_____

_____

OIL NAME

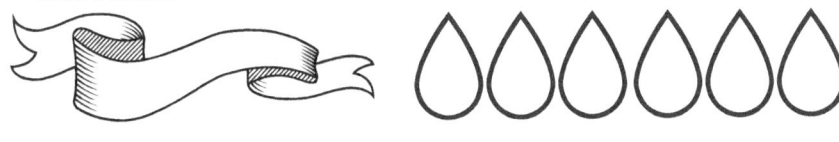

BENEFITS

_____

_____

_____

NOTES

_____

_____

_____

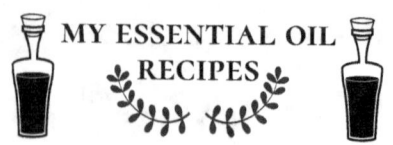

MY ESSENTIAL OIL RECIPES

OIL NAME

BENEFITS

_____

_____

_____

_____

NOTES

_____

_____

_____

_____

OIL NAME

BENEFITS

_____

_____

_____

_____

NOTES

_____

_____

_____

_____

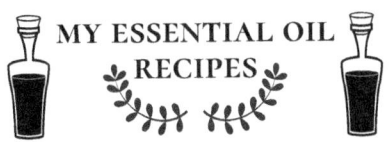

MY ESSENTIAL OIL RECIPES

OIL NAME

BENEFITS

_____

_____

_____

NOTES

_____

_____

_____

OIL NAME

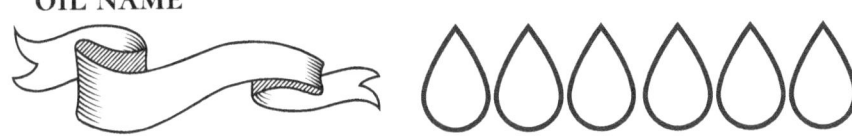

BENEFITS

_____

_____

_____

NOTES

_____

_____

_____

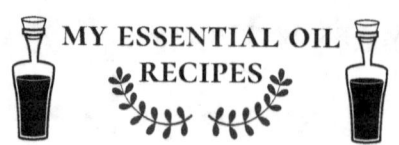

MY ESSENTIAL OIL RECIPES

OIL NAME

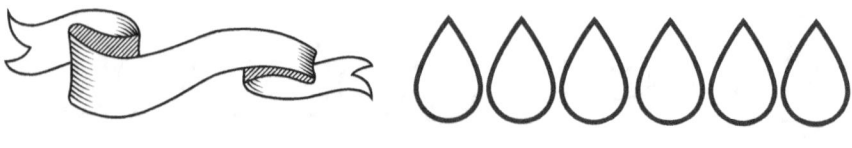

BENEFITS

_____

_____

_____

_____

NOTES

_____

_____

_____

_____

OIL NAME

BENEFITS

_____

_____

_____

_____

NOTES

_____

_____

_____

_____

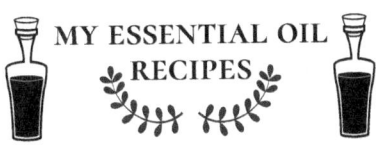

MY ESSENTIAL OIL RECIPES

OIL NAME

BENEFITS

_____

_____

_____

NOTES

_____

_____

_____

OIL NAME

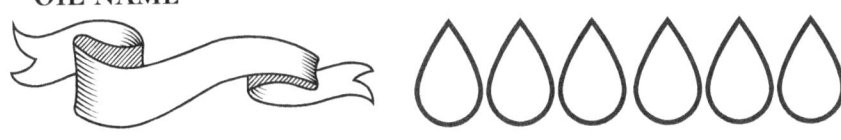

BENEFITS

_____

_____

_____

NOTES

_____

_____

_____

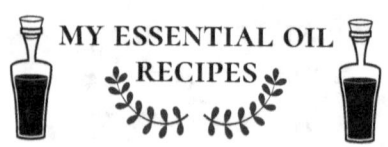

MY ESSENTIAL OIL RECIPES

OIL NAME

BENEFITS

_____

_____

_____

_____

NOTES

_____

_____

_____

_____

OIL NAME

BENEFITS

_____

_____

_____

_____

NOTES

_____

_____

_____

_____

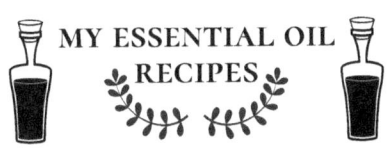

MY ESSENTIAL OIL RECIPES

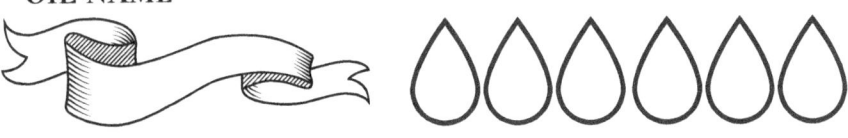

OIL NAME

BENEFITS

_____

_____

_____

NOTES

_____

_____

_____

OIL NAME

BENEFITS

_____

_____

_____

NOTES

_____

_____

_____

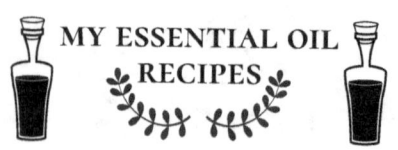

MY ESSENTIAL OIL RECIPES

OIL NAME

BENEFITS

_____

_____

_____

_____

NOTES

_____

_____

_____

_____

OIL NAME

BENEFITS

_____

_____

_____

_____

NOTES

_____

_____

_____

_____

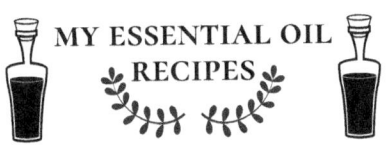

MY ESSENTIAL OIL RECIPES

OIL NAME

BENEFITS

NOTES

OIL NAME

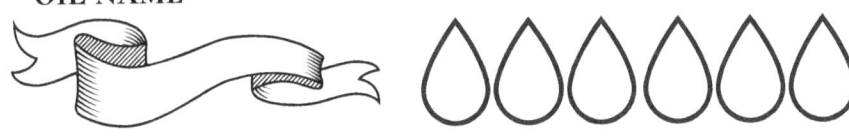

BENEFITS

NOTES

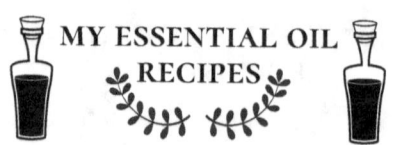

MY ESSENTIAL OIL RECIPES

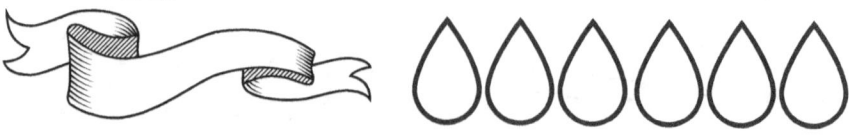

OIL NAME

BENEFITS

_____

_____

_____

_____

NOTES

_____

_____

_____

OIL NAME

BENEFITS

_____

_____

_____

_____

NOTES

_____

_____

_____

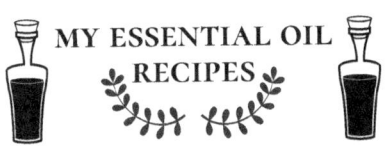

MY ESSENTIAL OIL RECIPES

OIL NAME

BENEFITS

NOTES

OIL NAME

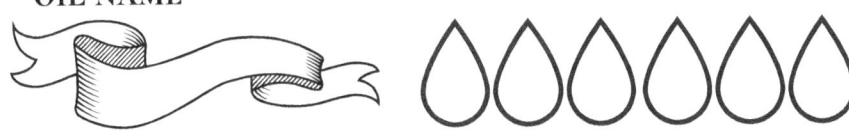

BENEFITS

NOTES

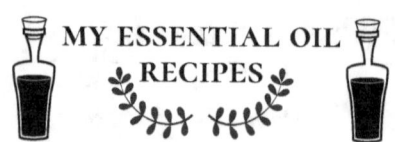

MY ESSENTIAL OIL RECIPES

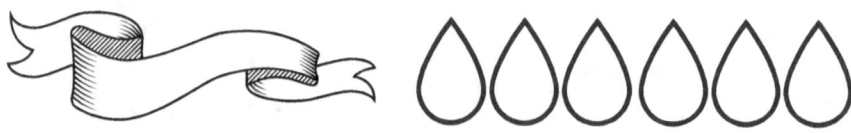

OIL NAME

BENEFITS

_____

_____

_____

_____

NOTES

_____

_____

_____

_____

OIL NAME

BENEFITS

_____

_____

_____

_____

NOTES

_____

_____

_____

_____

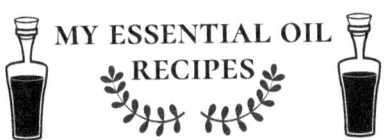

MY ESSENTIAL OIL RECIPES

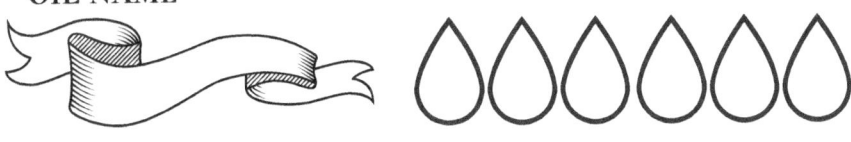

OIL NAME

BENEFITS

_____

_____

_____

_____

NOTES

_____

_____

_____

OIL NAME

BENEFITS

_____

_____

_____

_____

NOTES

_____

_____

_____

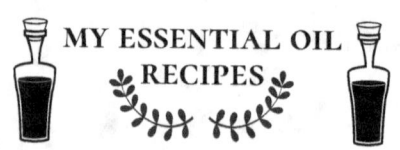

MY ESSENTIAL OIL RECIPES

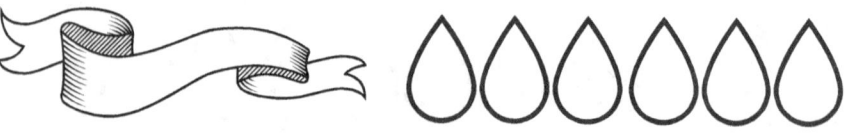

OIL NAME

BENEFITS

_____

_____

_____

_____

NOTES

_____

_____

_____

OIL NAME

BENEFITS

_____

_____

_____

_____

NOTES

_____

_____

_____

_____

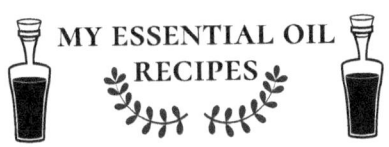

MY ESSENTIAL OIL RECIPES

OIL NAME

BENEFITS

_____
_____
_____
_____

NOTES

_____
_____
_____

OIL NAME

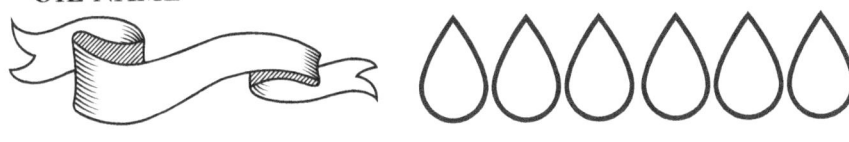

BENEFITS

_____
_____
_____
_____

NOTES

_____
_____
_____

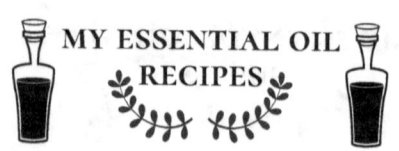

MY ESSENTIAL OIL RECIPES

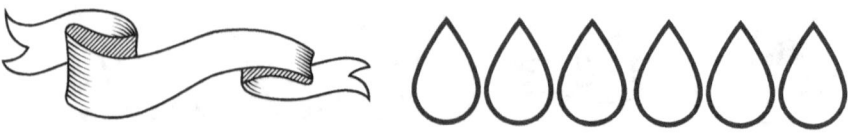

OIL NAME

BENEFITS

_____

_____

_____

_____

NOTES

_____

_____

_____

_____

OIL NAME

BENEFITS

_____

_____

_____

_____

NOTES

_____

_____

_____

_____

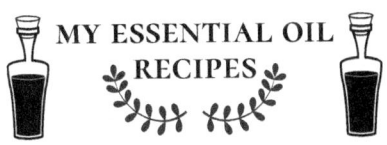

MY ESSENTIAL OIL RECIPES

OIL NAME

BENEFITS

NOTES

OIL NAME

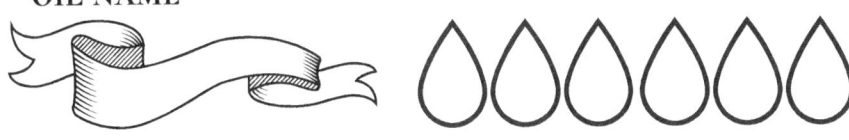

BENEFITS

NOTES

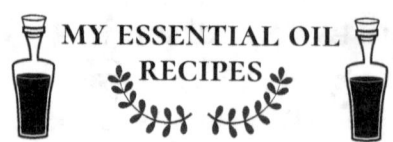

MY ESSENTIAL OIL RECIPES

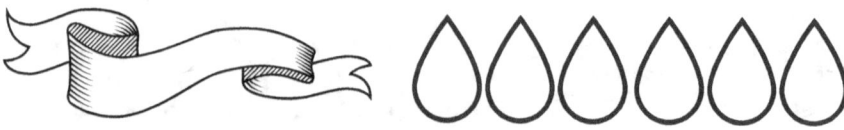

OIL NAME

BENEFITS

_____
_____
_____
_____

NOTES

_____
_____
_____
_____

OIL NAME

BENEFITS

_____
_____
_____
_____

NOTES

_____
_____
_____
_____

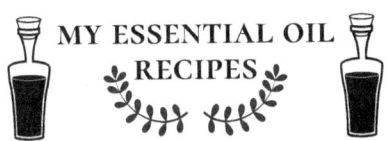

MY ESSENTIAL OIL RECIPES

OIL NAME

BENEFITS

_____

_____

_____

_____

NOTES

_____

_____

_____

_____

OIL NAME

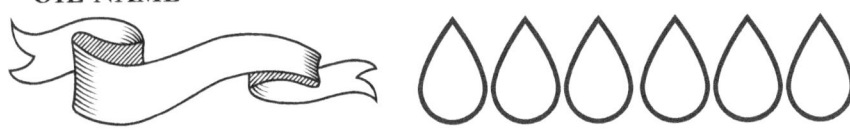

BENEFITS

_____

_____

_____

_____

NOTES

_____

_____

_____

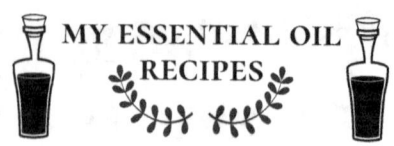

MY ESSENTIAL OIL RECIPES

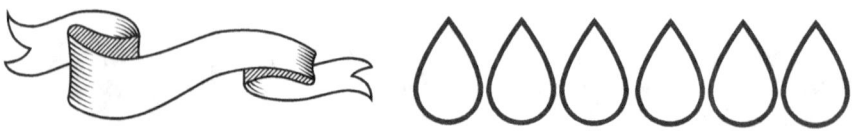

OIL NAME

BENEFITS

_____

_____

_____

_____

NOTES

_____

_____

_____

OIL NAME

BENEFITS

_____

_____

_____

_____

NOTES

_____

_____

_____

_____

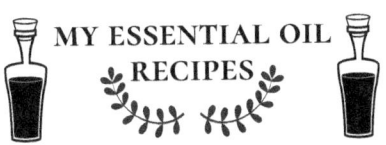

MY ESSENTIAL OIL RECIPES

OIL NAME

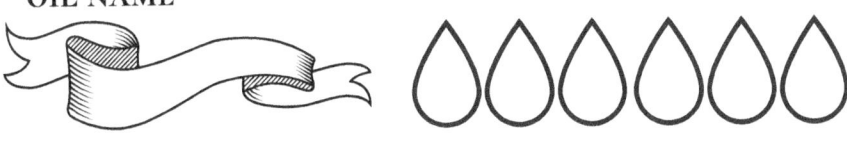

BENEFITS

_____

_____

_____

NOTES

_____

_____

_____

OIL NAME

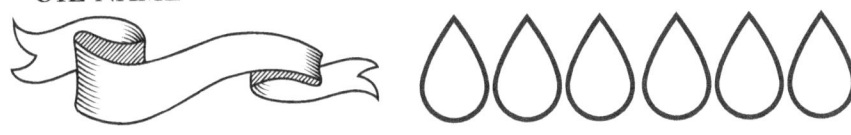

BENEFITS

_____

_____

_____

NOTES

_____

_____

_____

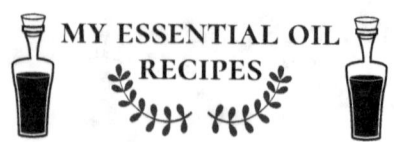

MY ESSENTIAL OIL RECIPES

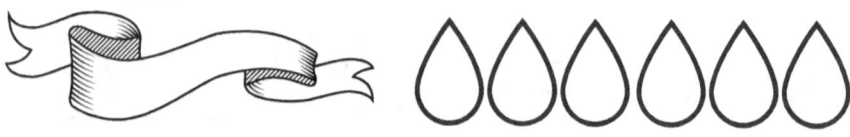

OIL NAME

BENEFITS

_____

_____

_____

_____

NOTES

_____

_____

_____

OIL NAME

BENEFITS

_____

_____

_____

_____

NOTES

_____

_____

_____

_____

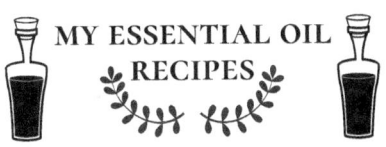

MY ESSENTIAL OIL RECIPES

OIL NAME

BENEFITS

_____

_____

_____

NOTES

_____

_____

_____

OIL NAME

BENEFITS

_____

_____

_____

NOTES

_____

_____

_____

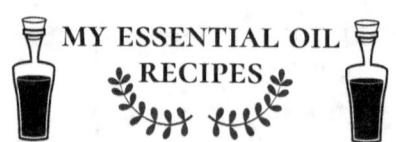

MY ESSENTIAL OIL RECIPES

OIL NAME

BENEFITS

_____

_____

_____

_____

NOTES

_____

_____

_____

_____

OIL NAME

BENEFITS

_____

_____

_____

_____

NOTES

_____

_____

_____

_____

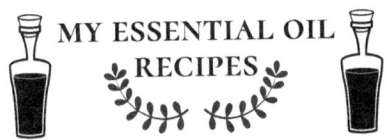

MY ESSENTIAL OIL RECIPES

OIL NAME

BENEFITS

_____

_____

_____

_____

NOTES

_____

_____

_____

_____

OIL NAME

BENEFITS

_____

_____

_____

_____

NOTES

_____

_____

_____

_____

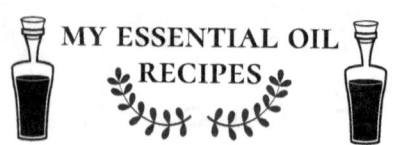

MY ESSENTIAL OIL RECIPES

OIL NAME

BENEFITS

_____

_____

_____

_____

NOTES

_____

_____

_____

_____

OIL NAME

BENEFITS

_____

_____

_____

_____

NOTES

_____

_____

_____

_____

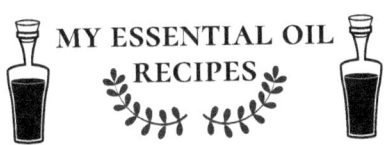

MY ESSENTIAL OIL RECIPES

OIL NAME

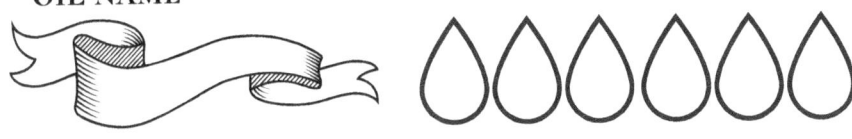

BENEFITS

_____

_____

_____

_____

NOTES

_____

_____

_____

_____

OIL NAME

BENEFITS

_____

_____

_____

_____

NOTES

_____

_____

_____

_____

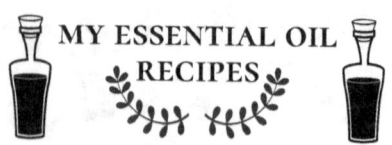

MY ESSENTIAL OIL RECIPES

OIL NAME

BENEFITS

_____
_____
_____
_____

NOTES

_____
_____
_____
_____

OIL NAME

BENEFITS

_____
_____
_____
_____

NOTES

_____
_____
_____
_____

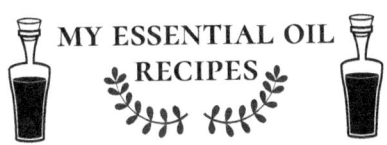

MY ESSENTIAL OIL RECIPES

OIL NAME

BENEFITS

_____

_____

_____

NOTES

_____

_____

_____

_____

OIL NAME

BENEFITS

_____

_____

_____

NOTES

_____

_____

_____

_____

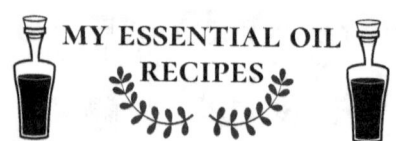

MY ESSENTIAL OIL RECIPES

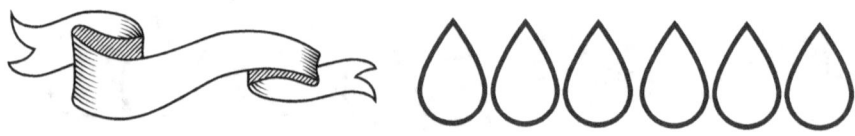

OIL NAME

BENEFITS

_____

_____

_____

_____

NOTES

_____

_____

_____

OIL NAME

BENEFITS

_____

_____

_____

_____

NOTES

_____

_____

_____

_____

www.ingramcontent.com/pod-product-compliance
Lightning Source LLC
Chambersburg PA
CBHW072107280526
45788CB00006B/2429